SPEECH AND LANGUAGE DISORDERS

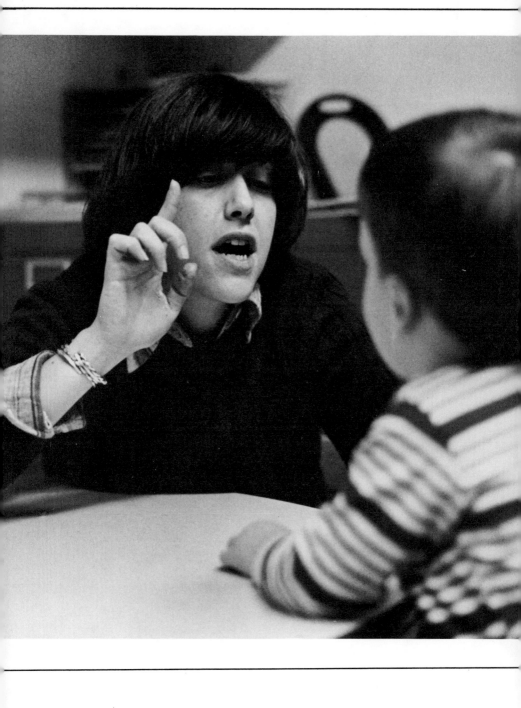

SPEECH AND LANGUAGE DISORDERS

BY GILDA BERGER

A GROLIER COMPANY

FRANKLIN WATTS
New York/London/Toronto/Sydney/1981
AN IMPACT BOOK

Diagrams by Vantage Art, Inc.

Photographs courtesy of Mimi Forsyth/Monk-
meyer Press Photo Service; p. ii; New York Pub-
lic Library Picture Collection: pp. 3, 5, and 12;
Hugh Rogers/Monkmeyer Press Photo Service:
pp. 31, 38, and 71; Lexington School for the
Deaf: p. 35; Irene B. Bayer/Monkmeyer Press
Photo Service: p. 37; Monkmeyer Press Photo
Service: p. 64.

Library of Congress
Cataloging in Publication Data

Berger, Gilda.
    Speech and language disorders.

    (An Impact book)
    Bibliography: p.
    Includes index.
    SUMMARY: Explains how we speak and
examines various problems involved in speaking and how they can be overcome.
    1. Speech, Disorders of—Juvenile liter-
ature. 2. Language disorders—Juvenile literature. [1. Speech—Disorders. 2. Speech therapy]
I. Title.
RC423.B44   616.85′5   80–27235
ISBN 0–531–04263–4

CONTENTS

7023777

CHAPTER 1.
The Origins of Speech
1

CHAPTER 2.
What Are Speech and Language Disorders?
7

CHAPTER 3.
The Apparatus for Speech
10

CHAPTER 4.
From Making Sounds to Using Words
22

CHAPTER 5.
Speech Errors
30

CHAPTER 6.
Stuttering
41

CHAPTER 7.
Unpleasant Voices
49

CHAPTER 8.
Language Difficulties
57

CHAPTER 9.
Multiple Difficulties
68

Glossary
77

Speech Organizations
81

Bibliography
82

Suggested Reading
83

Index
85

SPEECH AND LANGUAGE DISORDERS

CHAPTER 1.

THE ORIGINS OF SPEECH

Spoken language seems a natural part of our world. It is hard to even imagine a world without human speech.

Yet there was a time when people did not speak. Human beings have been around for approximately two million years. There is little likelihood that early humans used words. Although we don't know when language first appeared, we know it took hundreds of thousands of years to develop.

We will probably never know just when or where people first learned to talk. Evidence of early human speech is very hard to find. It cannot be dug out of the ground or discovered carved or painted on stone. The clues that we do find come to us only indirectly.

Archaeologists have unearthed many remnants of pre-historic civilizations. On occasion they have found complex structures from the past made of huge timbers. These

1

buildings suggest groups of people working together. Co-operation implies some kind of communication.

Imagine that you wanted to build a house. How would you get others to help you? How would you let them know that you wanted them to chop trees for lumber? How could you get others to understand that if they helped you build your house, you would help them build what they wanted? For communication and cooperation to take place, you need language.

Many burial sites from prehistoric times suggest that the people practiced some sort of religion. Religious activity usually indicates the presence of language. However, the actual words that were used, the prayers and chants, may never be known.

Some anthropologists and psychologists look for clues to the origin of language in the behavior of today's chimpanzees and gorillas. Fossil remains seem to show that we are descended from a line of development that branched off from the apes several million years ago.

Chimpanzees have been brought into homes and raised like human children. Even after years of careful training, however, the apes could still say only a few words.

We now think that the difficulty may be anatomical. The lower jaw of an ape closely resembles the lower jaw of a newborn baby. The throat is too narrow and rigid to make most sounds. And an ape does not normally use its lips or tongue to form sounds.

Humans and apes may share a common ancestor, but at some point the two lines split off, and the ancestors of humans began to walk erect, use tools, and develop speech.

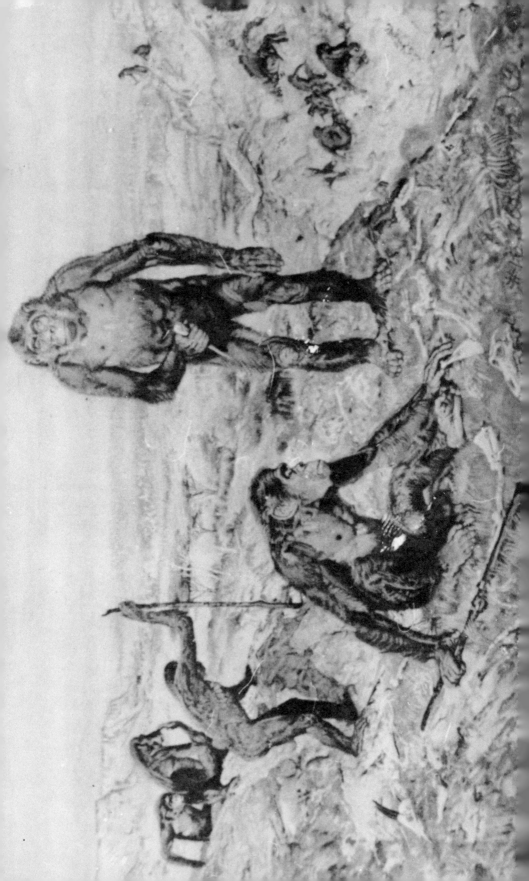

Some scientists have tried to teach apes to speak by sign language rather than by vocal means. The apes have mastered hundreds of different hand signals. They are now learning to send and receive messages by means of computerized "talking typewriters."

What does this tell us? Some believe it shows that apes can use language. Others insist that apes are merely imitating their human trainers. Even those who believe that apes use language, though, do not believe that they communicate like humans.

The part of the brain that is considered the source of speech is very tiny in the chimpanzee and gorilla. This same part is also very small in the fossil brain of very early humans. We don't know how large a brain must be to be capable of speech, but we do know that a child does not learn to speak until its brain has grown larger than that of the first humans. Therefore, it is believed that the first people to speak had a brain size at least as large as that of a one-year-old child.

The first people were probably stalkers of wild animals. Gradually they turned from stalking to hunting prey. To be good hunters, they needed to be able to communicate by sound with other hunters. They also needed the ability to solve problems quickly and to interpret the gestures of others. One theory on the origin of speech holds that air from the lungs, forced out while the hunter was running, became cries and yells. Repetition or imitation of these sounds eventually established

The chimpanzee Lana "talks" by using a computer keyboard at the Yerkes Primate Research Center in Atlanta, Georgia.

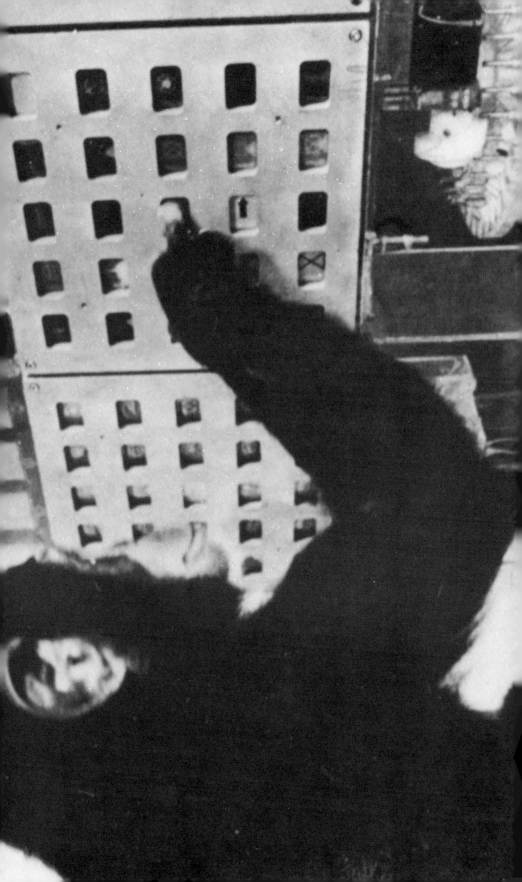

them as words. Then, according to this theory, simple vocabulary came into being. These first words became the basis for spoken language.

Language begins when two or more individuals agree to attach the same meaning to the same sounds. They use these sounds over and over again, with the meanings that have been attached to them. The meanings are symbols that stand for objects, actions, feelings, or ideas. With these symbols we are able to communicate with other human beings.

Our culture grew and developed as people talked to each other and passed their knowledge on to their children. Without language for communication, there would be little or no science, art, literature, or philosophy.

Whatever its origin, speech was and still is an activity that needs to be learned. It is a uniquely human tool. It played an important part in the evolution of humanity from its earliest beginnings, and it continues to play an important part in the growth and development of every one of us today.

CHAPTER 2.

WHAT ARE SPEECH AND LANGUAGE DISORDERS?

"Alex," the teacher called out, "who is the composer of the opera *Carmen*?"

At the sound of his name, Alex ducked his head down and clenched his hands into fists. After a few seconds he looked up, his face screwed into a frown.

"I think it's ..." A long silence followed. Then Alex began again. "I think it's ... B–B–B–Bizet."

Alex tried not to notice the teacher's look of pity, nor pay attention to his classmates' stifled giggles.

"I wa ambo wd fye," Sara told the waitress.

The waitress shook her head. Sara repeated her order, but to no avail.

"I'm sorry, I just can't understand you," the waitress said. "Tell me again, what do you want?"

Sara tried once more, a little louder. But the waitress shrugged her shoulders. Exasperated, Sara opened the menu and pointed to the desired item.

"Oh, why didn't you say so?" said the waitress. "One hamburger and fries coming up."

"Bus . . . shop cent?" Janet asked the bus driver in a timid voice.

"What did you say?" the bus driver asked.

"I want . . . bus . . . shop cent," Janet replied.

"You want to go to the shopping center?" the driver asked.

Janet nodded.

"OK, come on in. It's the last stop."

These stories illustrate just a few of the many speech disorders that afflict people. Most of us do not realize how widespread such problems are. According to one government report, about ten million Americans, or one out of every twenty people, suffer from a speech disorder.

Among school-aged children alone, over two million have serious speech difficulties and need special help. When we include people with speech problems resulting from hearing loss, the number is even greater. Altogether about twenty million persons, including four million children, suffer some sort of difficulty due to a speech, language, or hearing problem.

A speech disorder is usually thought of as any defect that makes a person's speech difficult to understand. People with speech disorders call attention to themselves because of the way they speak. They are always being asked to repeat what they have said. "What was that?" "Could you say that again?" "Please speak a little louder." These are the familiar comments heard daily by speech-disordered individuals.

Those with articulation disorders have difficulty

making sounds accurately and stringing them together easily. They may substitute one sound for another (*fun* for *sun*) or omit a sound (*ba* for *bat*). Stutterers suffer an interruption in the flow or rhythm of speech. They may involuntarily stop (May I have a . . . carrot, please?), repeat a sound (I need t–t–t–ten cents), or prolong a sound (He ra–a–a–an home). And individuals with voice disorders have inappropriate pitch (too low, too high, or monotonous), inappropriate volume (too loud or too soft), or poor voice quality (too harsh, hoarse, or breathy).

People with language disorders are unable to use the sounds of speech or words properly. They may say *hopsital* instead of *hospital* or jumble up meanings and say, for example, *breakfast* when they mean *supper*.

Finally, there are those who have a combination of articulation, voice, and language difficulties. Often, in these cases, some physical disability that was present at birth interferes with the speech or language-learning process.

Few of us speak perfectly. All of us sometimes experience difficulties in communication. And there are many normal variations in our abilities to articulate the sounds of speech and put our thoughts into words. But these differences are only considered disorders when they interfere with the way we express ourselves and the way we learn, in school or out.

9

CHAPTER 3.

THE APPARATUS FOR SPEECH

Speech is the way we produce sounds that others understand as words. Language is our ability to use speech sounds to express thoughts and emotions.

We need words in order to think and talk. We need words, or language, to express our ideas, share our feelings, make known our wants and needs, and have meaningful relationships with family and friends.

Ours is an intensely verbal society. About ninety percent of all human communication takes place through spoken language. Each of us speaks approximately five thousand words every day.

We depend on our ability to communicate with others. When we are near others who do not speak or understand what we say, as in a foreign country, we realize how vital words are to our existence.

When the Spanish explorers first reached the southeastern part of Mexico in the early sixteenth century, they asked the Indians the name of their homeland. The Indians answered "Yucatan," and so that's what the Spaniards named the new land. But, in fact, the Indians had not understood the question. In the Indians' language, *Yucatan* means "What do you want?"

People with speech disorders in our society are a little like the Spaniards arriving in Mexico for the first time. They are not understood and are somewhat out of touch with the world they live in. Some find it hard to make friends or fit in, even with family members. At school, the person may find it very difficult to keep up with the work. And when it is time to get and hold a job, there is discrimination to be faced. People with serious speech disorders often earn their living in a way that is below their potential.

People with speech defects may be teased, laughed at, or rejected. Stutterers are often made fun of, people who lisp are frequently ridiculed, and youngsters who speak in very high- or very low-pitched voices may be shunned.

One fourteen-year-old boy who stutters says that he is always being told to "speak up like a man." When that happens, he withdraws and becomes very quiet. He needs a part-time job but finds it hard to get one. He'd like to go out with a girl in school but he is afraid to call her up. This boy is growing cold and distant. Eventually his emotional problems may become more of a handicap than the speech disorder itself.

To be sure, there are many examples of individuals who have overcome speech disorders to become great successes. The Hebrew prophet Moses and the Greek orator Demosthenes are good examples from ancient times. Although Moses stuttered, it did not stop him from leading the Israelites out of Egypt, pleading with

11

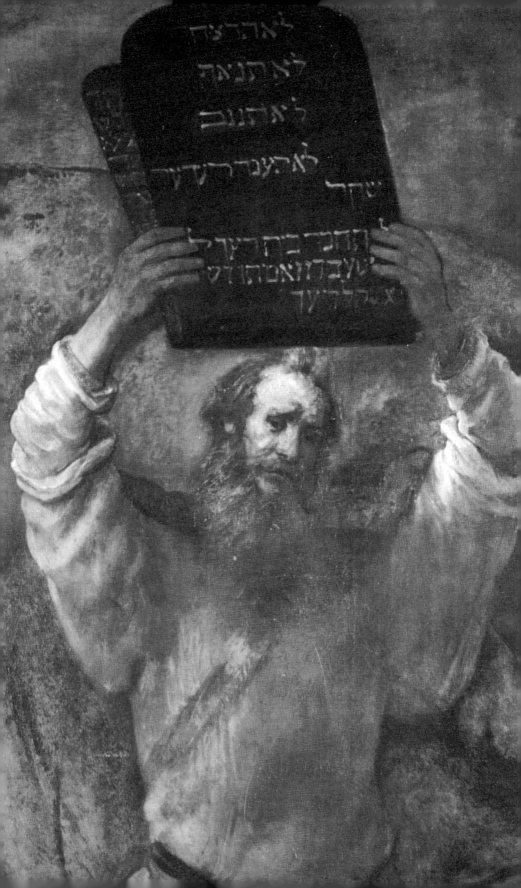

the Lord on Mt. Sinai, and taking his people to the promised land. Demosthenes overcame a rough, unpleasant voice and an awkward manner to become famous for arguing Greek law and politics in public. It is said that he improved his speech by reciting as he climbed steep hills and shouting above the roar of the ocean with a mouth full of pebbles.

Yet, though there are exceptions, for most people a severe speech defect is frustrating and disabling.

THE WAY WE SPEAK

Speaking and communicating with others involves three functions: producing sound, receiving sound, and interpreting sound. Speech disorders can arise from difficulties in any or all of these three areas.

When you talk, you produce sound. Sounds are made by setting an object into a rapid back-and-forth motion called vibration. Speaking forces air from the lungs up through the windpipe, or trachea, and out past the voice box, or larynx. In the larynx, the moving air sets two small bands of tissue, called the vocal cords, or, more properly, the vocal folds, into vibration.

The vibrating vocal folds produce a low-pitched buzzing sound. This sound is the basic raw material of speech. Many things happen to the basic sound as it passes through the vocal tract.

Tensing the vocal folds makes them shorter and causes the pitch of the sound to go up. Relaxing the folds makes them longer, and the pitch goes down. Greater air

Moses, known to have had a speech impediment, is displaying the Ten Commandments in this painting by Rembrandt.

pressure on the folds makes the sound louder; less pressure produces a softer sound. Altogether the vocal cords can assume about 170 different positions!

Above the larynx is a passageway, called the pharynx, which opens into the nose and mouth. The walls of the pharynx, and also the soft palate, tongue, lips, and jaws, are all able to move. As these so-called articulators change position, they further alter the sound coming from the larynx.

Say a simple word like "church." Can you detect some of the movements that formed the sounds? You can say the word because your vocal folds and articulators are able to make the twenty or so different adjustments that are needed. Since it takes less than one-fourth of a second to say "church," each movement can take no more than one-eightieth of a second. Good speech, then, is made by controlling many tiny movements that must occur rapidly and in a precise way and certain order.

No matter how well you made sounds, though, you could not be heard without some sort of amplifying equipment. The chest, throat, nose, sinuses, and mouth all act as resonators. They produce louder sounds than those made by the vocal folds. The chest adds resonance to low-pitched sounds. The nose and sinuses amplify most higher-pitched tones. And the throat and mouth add resonance to almost the entire range of pitches used in speech.

Any difficulty along the vocal tract can produce speech that is slurred, unpleasant, or hard to understand. When you cannot coordinate your muscles or control your breathing, you cannot make the correct sounds. When you cannot move your tongue, lips, or jaws, you cannot shape sound into words.

THE WAY WE HEAR

When you produce a sound, you set the air near your mouth into vibration. This starts a sort of chain reac-

14

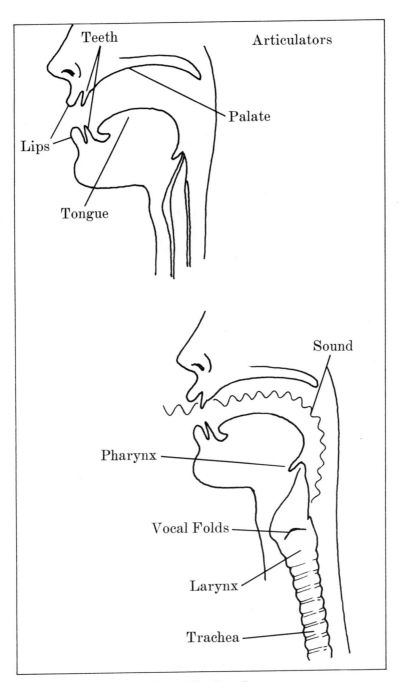

How We Speak

tion, with each molecule of air bumping into a nearby molecule and causing that molecule, in turn, to vibrate. The vibrations spread out in all directions in a wavelike motion.

Sound waves enter the outer ear and are channeled through the hearing canal to the eardrum, or tympanic membrane. The membrane is like a skin stretched over a drum. A sound passing down the ear canal causes the membrane to vibrate.

On the other side of the eardrum is the middle ear, an air-filled cavity that contains a chain of three tiny bones: the hammer, anvil, and stirrup. These bones modify the sound (amplify soft sounds and soften loud ones) and then pass the vibrations from the tympanic membrane along to the inner ear.

The inner ear chamber is filled with a fluid. Sound enters the inner ear through an opening called the oval window and sets this fluid in motion. Special cells in the cochlea, a spiral-shaped structure in the lower portion of the inner ear, "feel" the movements of the fluid. This triggers the nerve endings to send electrical signals, by way of the auditory nerve, to the hearing centers of the brain, where the signals are perceived as sound.

Hearing is essential to the way we produce sounds as well as the way we receive speech. We speak as we hear. When someone cannot hear clearly, he or she cannot distinguish among sounds and therefore cannot learn to say the sounds correctly. This difficulty in distinguishing among sounds can also make it hard to express thoughts and master language.

THE WAY WE INTERPRET SOUND
The nerve signals from the ears reach the brain as an electrical code. The brain deciphers the code according to its stored memory and understanding of all the

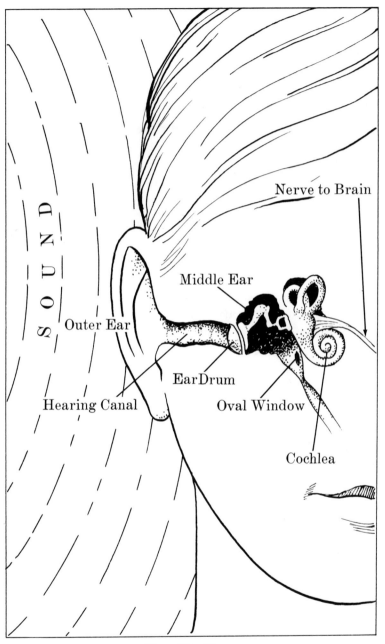

S O U N D

Nerve to Brain

Middle Ear

Outer Ear

Ear Drum

Hearing Canal

Oval Window

Cochlea

How We Hear

sounds heard since birth. Nerve pathways connect the brain's memory center with other areas in the brain that control muscle movement and thought. An injury to or disease in any of these areas of the brain can cause nerve loss. Loss of hearing, loss of speech, or paralysis of certain muscles may follow an injury to the brain.

What flashes through your mind when you hear the word *elephant?* A four-legged animal with a trunk, of course. At the sound of the word, you visualize an elephant. You do this because your brain is able to associate the sound of the word with a visual memory of an elephant. The auditory center in your brain connects the sounds you hear with their meanings.

Different parts of your brain cooperate in the same way when you think *elephant* and then say the word out loud. You use the muscles of your lips and tongue to make the sounds. Control of these muscles comes from the motor speech part of the brain working together with the auditory speech center. In other words, the brain coordinates the faculties of speech and hearing.

Some individuals are not able to make the needed associations between different parts of the brain. Thus, they may not be able to understand the meanings of the sounds they hear. They may have difficulty understanding language. They may find it hard to express their thoughts in words. They may even find it hard to think in words.

Delayed language, or a marked slowness in the development of the skills needed for understanding and expressing thoughts and ideas, is the most common language disorder. It may result from brain damage. Children with learning disabilities usually have language disorders due to impaired ability to receive or express ideas.

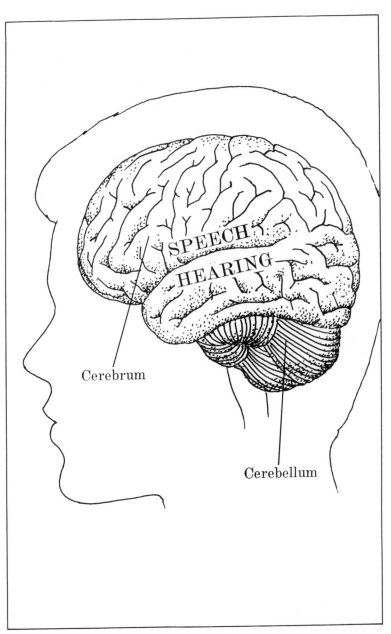

How We Interpret Sound

Disturbances in the way we speak, hear, and interpret what is said to us are not the only causes of speech problems. Language development begins early in life. It begins the first time we cry and get picked up to be cuddled or fed. Disturbances in the way we speak may result if there is a lack of affection early in life, not enough human contact, a poor environment, overprotective parents, or too much pressure to conform or achieve, among a number of other factors.

Human growth and the development of speech and language are highly complex processes. It is almost impossible, therefore, to find single causes for speech problems. Most experts now believe that such problems usually result from a combination of causes.

People with speech defects can and are being helped by speech experts. Such professionals are called speech-language pathologists by the American Speech-Language-Hearing Association. More commonly they are known as speech therapists, speech clinicians, or speech teachers.

There are many different ways to diagnose problems and determine treatment. Success often varies with the problem. Generally, though, the less severe the defect, the greater the chance of correcting faulty speech patterns.

Most speech therapists feel that the earlier a speech defect is diagnosed, the easier it is to treat. In the words of one therapist: "By the time we get to the person with a serious speech defect, it may take months just to get the person to admit that he or she has a problem." That's why it's important for all of us to learn how to recognize speech disabilities. The sooner such disorders are treated, the better the chances are of preventing them from becoming a lifelong handicap.

What are some signs of a speech or language disorder? Here are three that are very common:

• A person's speech or language is so different from others of the same age, sex, and ethnic group that it is difficult to understand and it attracts unfavorable attention.

• A person appears to have difficulty hearing or understanding the speech of others.

• A person avoids communicating with others because he or she is self-conscious about speaking, hearing, or language ability.

Anyone who exhibits these or other signs of a speech disorder should receive a thorough evaluation by a speech-language pathologist to determine the problem and begin a plan of treatment.

CHAPTER 4.

FROM MAKING SOUNDS TO USING WORDS

Most likely you rarely think about talking. You just do it. Talking is part of your everyday life, and you almost surely take it for granted. You may even forget, sometimes, that you were not born with speech. It didn't just come to you. You had to learn to speak.

You probably would not have learned to speak if you had not had contact with others who do. Children in institutions who grow up with little attention from adults are often slow to speak. Your parents, older brothers and sisters, and later your friends actually taught you to speak and to use language. Like every other human, you had to go through the stages of crying, babbling, repeating single words, and finally, of speaking in phrases, sentences, and whole thoughts.

Learning to talk, then, does not really come "naturally.'' The development of speech and language is a long, complex, and often difficult process.

CRIES AND COOS

Most people do not realize that children begin to learn to speak from the day they are born. With their first cries, infants tell the world they are hungry, wet, or frightened. These so-called discomfort sounds say, in effect, ''I want to be fed, cleaned up, or comforted.''

The adult who hears the cries comes over and feeds the baby, changes its diaper, or picks up and cuddles the infant. Usually the person also smiles and coos at the child. Within the first month, infants learn that they too can coo and make the so-called comfort sounds. They gurgle, sigh, and grunt with satisfaction as they are fed, diapered, or held. If you listen carefully to these comfort sounds, you will hear some of the vowels and consonants that are later used in speaking.

The most important thing, though, about both the cries and the coos is that they have a purpose and a meaning for the child. The baby learns that crying makes its needs known. For most children it also means that their needs will be met by a concerned adult. The need to make sounds and to have them bring pleasure form the foundation of language.

Crying is good and necessary for another reason— it lets babies practice making sounds. By exercising the muscles of its larynx and mouth, a baby learns to adjust its volume from loud to soft and to vary its pitch from high to low.

Some speech experts, though, say that too much crying may have damaging results. Children who spend a great deal of time crying during their early years often have speech problems when they grow up. It may be that they do not get enough practice making the sounds of speech during this early period. Most of the speech sounds are practiced not when the baby is crying but when it is happy. Some unpleasant, whining voices in adults have been traced back to excessive crying as babies.

BABBLING

Around the fourth month of life, though cooing and crying continue, infants take another step in speech development. They begin to babble. Babbling is simply the repetition of certain sounds. It is done just for the fun of making the sounds and hearing the results.

Most babbling takes place when babies are alone. The sounds are made softly or loudly, separately or strung together. By making and hearing the sounds, the baby learns to associate the movements of its tongue and mouth with the sounds heard. This association is needed for acquiring the sounds of speech. Through babbling, children master the complex muscle movements that will eventually combine individual sounds to form words.

Parents who show an interest in their children's verbal experiments help them with speech and language development. Experts find that children who grow up in unstimulating homes are often delayed in their development.

At about five or six months of age, the baby starts to use inflections while babbling. "Pah-poh do, buh?" the child says while the parent looks on in amazement. The child seems to be asking questions, giving commands, making statements, or expressing needs. Only the proper words are lacking. This kind of vocal play, which sounds like gibberish, is called lallation.

The inflections do have meaning. Vocalization begins to take on some of the expressiveness of true speech.

24

Lallation goes on not only when the child is alone but also with others. Some parents play along. When the child makes sounds at them, they make the same sounds back. This exchange gives the child the idea that one uses sounds to give messages and receive them and eventually turns sound-making into talking.

Children who never babble, or who suddenly stop babbling, are usually showing the first signs of abnormal speech or language development. Those with a severe hearing loss, for example, will often stop babbling at around six months of age. These babies can make sounds just like others with hearing, but because they cannot participate in the give-and-take of communication, they do not learn to speak.

GESTURES

Learning how to send and receive messages in sound is only part of the communication that takes place between parent and child. If you had been born into a family of Eskimos you would have learned to show affection by pressing noses together with people you liked. In Thailand, you would have learned to shake your head from side to side when you meant "yes."

In those cultures, as in our own, gestures are part of getting the message across to other people. These gestures are often used together with sounds. Certain gestures and sounds go together. They come to stand for certain things. For example, a mother extends her arms and says, "Upsy daisy!" The baby learns to associate these words with being picked up. The baby learns that certain other words and gestures go with feeding, diapering, bathing, and rocking.

Word-gesture combinations are thought to be the first meaningful exchanges of language between parent and child. If the same tone and gestures are consistently

25

used, the baby learns to associate them. A smile and a kiss along with words such as "good" and "wonderful" show approval. Shaking the head or waving a finger and saying "no, no" indicates disapproval.

FIRST WORDS

Around its first birthday a child usually utters its first word. First words vary from child to child. But no matter the baby's nationality, these first words are all pretty much the same. Usually they start with the "easy sounds"—/m/, /w/, /p/, /b/, or /k/. Young children in the United States and most of Europe call their mothers by the universal word "mama." In some countries the same words are used but with different meanings. For example, "baba" means grandmother to the Russians; Americans take it to mean that the baby wants to go "bye-bye."

Often, the first word is a word of command—"Mum" for "Give me milk"—or a word of recognition, like "doggie" for dog. Adults treat these sounds as though they are meaningful. They repeat and stress them. Babies catch on that these words are important. They come to understand that certain sounds stand for certain things. Using these sounds helps babies get what they want.

Almost always the first words are made up of sounds that were practiced earlier in babbling and in vocal play with adults. At first, words like "kaca" have a general meaning. They can mean a cracker or pretzel or anything else that is edible. "Doggie" can refer to a dog, cat, or stuffed animal. They are usually words that the child understands that adults have used often.

Most parents encourage their baby's early attempts to use words. They help their child to learn new words. When the child does not know a word, they supply it. Say a toddler calls every animal it sees "doggie." When the child seems old enough to tell the difference between a dog and a cat, the parent will give the new word, "cat." The adult might say, "Cat says 'meow-meow.'" Learning new words and their meanings also aids in the child's overall mental development.

Even when they know a few words, some one-year-olds use a type of vocal play called jargon. Jargon is a stream of unintelligible jabber. It has been described as "pretend" conversation. The child "talks" to its parents, to its toys, even to the furniture, never repeating the same syllables twice. As the child's vocabulary grows, it gradually gives up the meaningless sounds of jargon.

WORDS INTO SENTENCES

Children begin to combine words into phrases and simple sentences at around one-and-a-half to two years of age. To understand how great a leap this is, try speaking for an hour or so in single words alone. The stringing together of words brings the child to a new stage in language development.

At this point, the child still has a comparatively small vocabulary. First sentences have been described as telegraphic speech. You may hear a child of this age say, "See doggie," "Doggie eat," "Ball fall down," and so on.

By age two, most children are using compound as well as simple sentences: "Johnny go in car, get Daddy." They speak loudly because their voices are not yet under control. During their second year, most children are able to understand long sentences. They can follow complex commands such as "Get the book from the table, bring it to me, and sit down so I can read to you." If you point to a familiar object, they will be able to name it by themselves. Children of this age can imitate sen-

27

tences of several words. They will frequently remember a new word after having heard it just once.

The speech rhythm of two- and three-year-olds is often broken. They hesitate, stumble, stop, and start. "Give me my, uh, my . . . uh, my teddy." This happens because it is hard to put words together. To the very young child, adult speech often sounds rushed and continuous, like an unbroken chain of syllables. Children who "stutter" at this point should not be pressured to speak fluently. Such pressure, in fact, may damage the child's chances for acquiring fluency later on.

The third and fourth years of life are commonly the high points in speech and language development. At this age children start to use a feedback system. They listen to the sounds they make and compare them with the speech of others around them. You will often hear children of nursery school age actively working to improve their speech. They are trying to produce speech that is easier to understand, more under control, and more expressive.

Frequently, children at this age are able to tell you what they think and what they want. They understand much of what is said to them. They can use words in their vocabulary to make long sentences. They can recognize and name from pictures many familiar objects or activities.

By the time children begin school, most are comfortable with spoken language. They can follow the teacher's instructions, listen to stories and answer questions, receive information, and use simple reasoning. Most can express themselves well enough to ask questions, give information, make their needs known, tell stories, list events in proper order, make choices, and predict the outcome of certain events.

Five-year-olds generally understand speech and language in many different situations. If they are lucky, for the rest of their lives they will continue to increase their vocabulary and sharpen and improve their speech and language skills.

What are some signs of normal speech and language development in children? Here, in review, are four of the more important ones:

• At birth or soon after, the infant cries. During the first month it coos and gurgles as well. At three to six months it babbles. It develops a variety of sounds to make its different needs known.

• A one-year-old enjoys imitating sounds and using jargon. From one-and-a-half to two years of age, the child learns about a dozen words and is able to ask two-word questions, construct simple sentences, and follow simple requests.

• At three or four years of age, the child uses four- and five-word sentences and is able to produce most sounds.

• A five-year-old says almost all sounds correctly, has a clear voice, and is able to hear and understand almost all speech.

CHAPTER 5.

SPEECH ERRORS

MISTAKES IN ARTICULATION

Jeffrey is a first-grader who has problems in articulation. Unlike most seven-year-olds, Jeff is not able to make all the sounds of speech correctly. Either he substitutes incorrect sounds for correct ones or he leaves out certain sounds altogether. When Jeff says, "I wef my tote at koo," he means to say, "I left my coat at school."

Even Jeff's mother finds it hard to understand him. His teacher is concerned that Jeff may fall behind in his schoolwork or become a behavior problem.

Articulation disorders are the most common of all speech problems. They make up about three out of every five speech or language disabilities. More than four out of every five speech disorders in children are related to articulation.

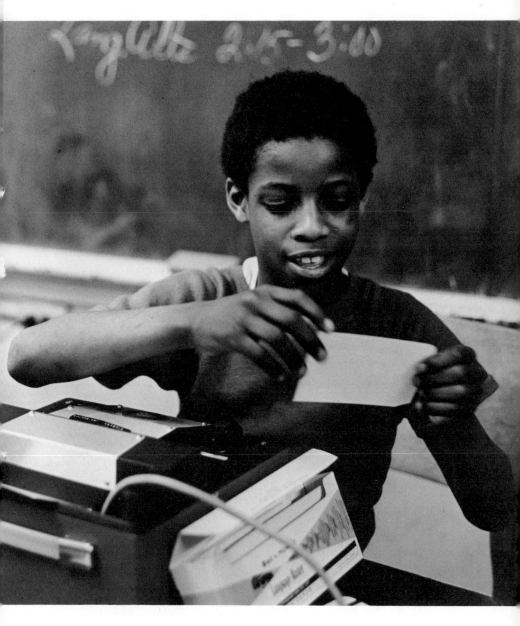

*Many kinds of tape and audio machines
are in use today in the treatment of
children with speech disabilities.*

Of course, if you were a king, an articulation disorder might not be much of a problem. According to the story, when King Philip II (1527–1598) of Spain wanted to say *ceilo* (sky), it came out *thielo*. And when he used the verb *decir* (to say), it sounded like *dethir*. Since the nobles always followed the patterns set by the king, they began to imitate his speech. For every /s/ they substituted /th/. The pronunciation spread and took hold in Spain. Even today, many people speak Spanish with an elegant lisp, saying "Barthelona" instead of "Barcelona," for example.

A lisp is an example of a substitution mistake. Errors of substitution occur more frequently than any other kind of articulation mistake. Although speakers can substitute any sound for the correct one, the most usual are /w/ for /r/ (*wain* for *rain*), /g/ for /c/ (*gat* for *cat*), and the lisp /th/ for /s/ (*thay* for *say*).

Almost as common are errors of omission. Omissions occur when no sound is produced for the correct sound. The speaker may say "bing" for "bring," "how" for "house," or "sell" for "settle."

Speech sounds are usually learned in a certain order. The simple sounds, such as /m/, /p/, /b/, and /t/, generally develop first. The more complicated sounds of /sh/, /ch/, /th/, and /z/ come later. The blends of consonants—/gr/, /cl/, /sp/, /tw/, and so on—are hardest to say correctly. That is why many seven-year-olds have trouble saying such words as "green," "clothing," and "spring." Some put in sounds that do not belong in the words. You may hear a vowel added between the /g/ and /r/ of "green," so that it comes out "guhreen." Or, a /k/ may be inserted into a word, resulting in "skun" instead of "sun."

And finally there is distortion in making speech sounds. The speaker may sound a little drunk or like someone who has just lost a few teeth. Distortions are substitutions of sounds that do not exist in our language for ones that do. A good example of distortion is excessive hissing on an /s/ sound.

Most children who start to talk around one year of age are using the correct sounds of speech by the time they are three. A few, of course, are not. The way adults react to speech errors in young children often determines how long the disorder will persist.

There are parents who believe that their children will outgrow articulation mistakes. They treat the substitutions, omissions, additions, or distortions of speech sounds as something "cute," or as "just baby talk." For these children, the mistakes tend to hang on.

Then, there are parents who harshly criticize or endlessly correct their children's speech. The children often dig in and refuse to change the way they speak. An approach that neither ignores nor overemphasizes the youngster's difficulties is usually best.

FINDING SPEECH ERRORS

Amy is a child who jabbered all the time but produced only a dozen or so words that were intelligible. She had just passed her sixth birthday when her parents brought her to a clinic for a speech, language, and hearing evaluation.

The speech-language pathologist started by taking Amy's developmental history. She was looking for clues to the origin of the speech defect. She questioned Amy's parents carefully.

A very important part of tracking down the cause of a disorder can be the medical examination. The physician will try to discover if the disorder is organic (stemming from a physical cause) or functional (due to another cause).

Since good hearing is essential to good speech, Amy was given a hearing test by a clinical audiologist. The clinician used an audiometer, a machine that produces pure sound at different pitches and varying levels of loudness. During the tests, Amy wore earphones. She was told to raise her hand when the sound was audible and lower her hand when she could no longer hear it. Both ears were tested, each one separately.

Once the hearing test was over, articulation tests were given to pinpoint her speech errors. One of the most popular group of tests was used, the Templin-Darley Articulation Tests. Amy was asked to say aloud the names of different objects. The pathologist kept a record of the girl's articulation of the test sounds. Later she spoke informally with Amy, asking her to repeat certain sentences, to count, and to name colors and the days of the week. She then prepared a list of the articulation errors Amy had made.

Malformations of the mouth or teeth and hearing loss are not the only causes of articulation errors. Neuro-muscular disabilities, such as cerebral palsy, can make it difficult to move the muscles of the face. This can lead to mistakes with certain sounds. Poor contact between the lips and teeth can cause errors with other sounds.

Articulation errors may also stem from faulty learning of the sounds of speech. Just why this happens is usually very difficult to determine. Sometimes parents who have poor speech set unsatisfactory models for their children. Parents with severe hearing disabili-

Audiometric testing can reveal hearing impairments even in very young children.

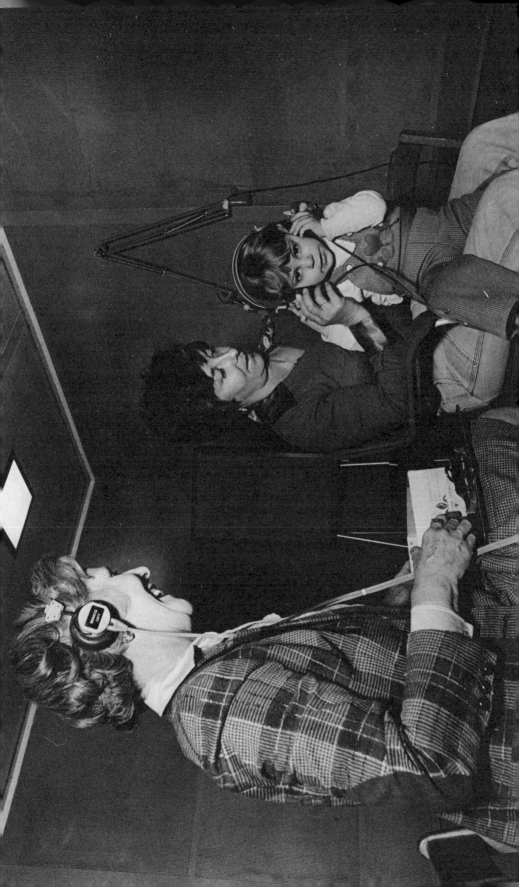

ties or who are foreign-speaking may also make it more difficult for young children to learn the correct sounds of speech.

CORRECTING ERRORS

Once the speech therapist decided that Amy could be helped to speak better, a treatment program was planned. Treatment can involve a number of different strategies. Sometimes an organic problem needs to be corrected before speech therapy can begin. If indifference or too much pressure by parents is involved, a psychologist may be called on to help improve the home situation. In Amy's case, speech therapy was begun at once. Two years later, Amy's speech was entirely understandable.

All errors in articulation can be helped. The most important factor, though, in the success of the therapy is always the child's readiness to change. Therefore, speech treatment usually begins by making the youngster aware of his or her articulation disorder.

If there are several errors, each one is treated separately, with concentration on only one at a time. The therapist usually starts by selecting the sound that is either used the most, that is the simplest to say, or that is acquired earliest in normal speech development.

First, the pathologist makes the child aware of the incorrect sound. The child may be asked to listen to correct and incorrect articulations of the sound and to differentiate between them. "Clap your hands every time you hear the target sound," the clinician might say, or, "I'll make three sounds. You tell me which one you make mistakes on."

Copying the correct sound is an important part of many speech therapies.

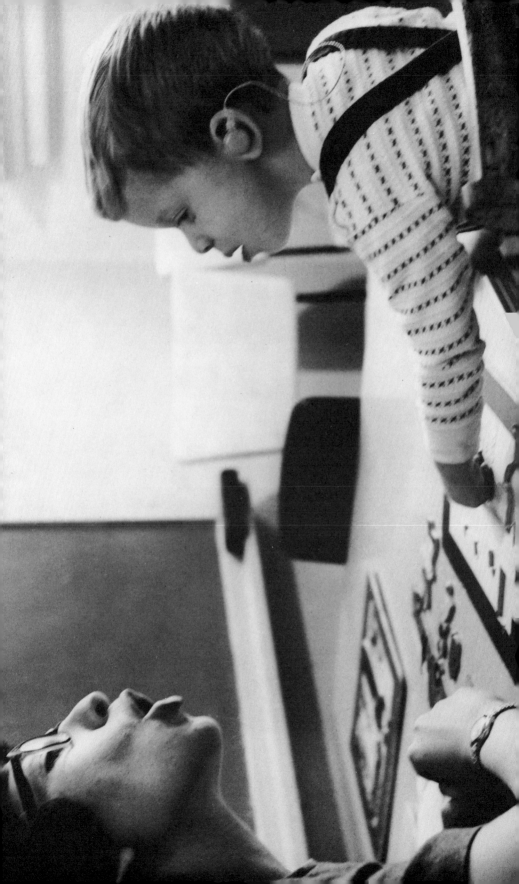

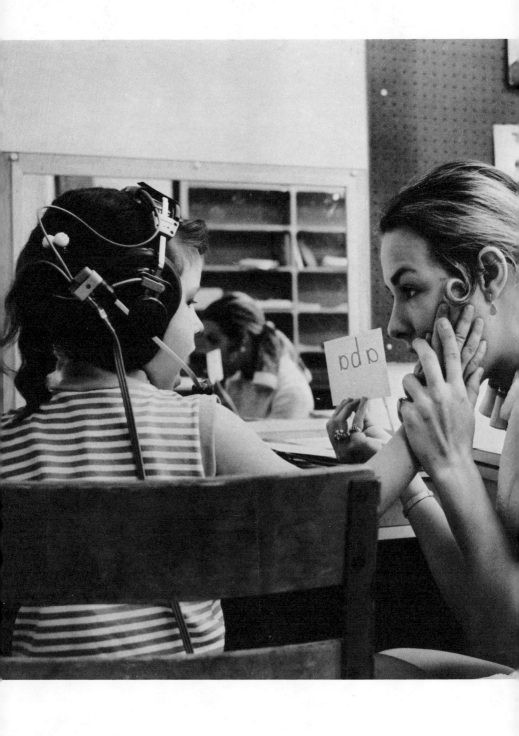

Once the child is able to isolate the incorrect sound, he or she is helped to "unlearn" the error and produce the correct sound. Prescribed exercises or games may build up the muscle coordination needed to make the new sounds. This may involve having the child say the sound approximately right, then repeating it over and over again, always trying to get closer to the exact sound. Or it may mean saying a similar sound, then modifying it until arriving at the correct sound.

After the sound is learned, it is used in a syllable, in a word, and finally in a full sentence. The aim of the therapy, no matter what strategy is used, is to help the person make the sound correctly and learn to use it in normal speech. Children are trained to listen to themselves and to catch and correct errors when they occur.

A number of speech teachers favor the sensory-motor approach. Here children are taught to be aware of the movements and positions of all parts of the throat and mouth while making sounds. The teacher can then focus on the development of proper sound-making in a step-by-step way.

Sometimes a system of rewards for following correct procedures, called operant conditioning, is used. The person is rewarded for making correct sounds or using sounds in the right way. The purpose is to help individuals acquire and strengthen new speech habits

At a speech and hearing clinic in Dallas, Texas, some children are taught to memorize the actual positions and movements of the mouth and jawline during speech.

while giving up the old ones. Eventually the reward is no longer needed.

The success of any program, however, often depends on the severity of the disorder and the age of the individual. People with fewer than three or four articulation mistakes can progress quite fast. In general, second- and third-graders, and even pre-schoolers, seem to improve faster than teenagers.

CHAPTER 6.

STUTTERING

STRUGGLES OF STUTTERERS

"My n–a–a–a–me is . . . M–a–a–ark No–No–No–lan. I'm a–a–a–, I'm a ju–ju–ju–junior at Central High."

Sixteen-year-old Mark has the most common speech disorder among teenagers, stuttering. Mark hesitates and postpones saying certain words until he thinks he can get them out smoothly. Sometimes he opens his mouth and nothing comes out. Sometimes he avoids certain words and instead uses words that he knows he can say. Other times, he just trails off in mid-sentence, without ever finishing his thought.

Often, when Mark struggles to speak, he jerks his head, blinks his eyes, grimaces, and stiffens his body. At times, he even slaps himself on the face, to help get the words out. These physical actions used to help him say the words and sounds that gave him the most trouble.

41

Now, they no longer work very well, but Mark finds it hard to rid himself of the habit.

Perhaps worst of all are Mark's feelings about himself. He does not trust himself to make telephone calls, and he never answers the phone when it rings. He doesn't tell jokes or stories. Members of his family order for him at restaurants. When asked what it is like to live with his problem, Mark says: "Talking is just very hard work. Sometimes I want to stop talking altogether. I hate to see the embarrassment or stifled smiles on people's faces."

While many stutterers share Mark's frustration, there are a few who manage to laugh at their difficulties. Homer Bigart, the Pulitzer Prize-winning war correspondent, has a stutter. He tells the story of how everyone worried when he was supposed to meet King George VI of Great Britain, also a stutterer. Would the king think Mr. Bigart was making fun of him? "Luckily," the reporter said with a chuckle, "the king breezed by me and I wasn't called upon to talk."

ONSET AND OCCURRENCE

Mark is one among some two million stutterers in the United States, approximately one percent of the population. As with most people who stutter, Mark's problem began to develop when he was about eight years old. Many children stutter, but for most the problem disappears as they grow older. Two out of every five who stutter before they are five years old no longer stutter by the time they are ten. Four out of five of all children who stutter outgrow the disorder by adolescence. But for Mark the problem hung on.

As far as is known, stuttering strikes with the same frequency all kinds of people in all walks of life. Although it occurs in both civilized and primitive societies, there is some evidence that cultures emphasizing verbal skills have a higher incidence of stuttering.

For reasons that are not yet known, stuttering seems to be sex-linked. It affects four times as many males as females.

WHY PEOPLE STUTTER

Unlike most other speech defects, the cause of stuttering is still not known. A great deal of research has been done and is still going on today. Over the last fifty years, there have been more articles published on stuttering than on any other speech disorder. Yet the disorder remains a mystery.

We all know how it feels to hesitate or stumble in speech, how embarrassing it is to be at a complete loss for words or to have a word at the tip of the tongue but somehow be unable to get it out.

One of the most popular American presidents was Dwight D. Eisenhower. When interviewed in public, Eisenhower often hesitated and repeated himself. Many of his interruptions were like those associated with stuttering. What is important was that Eisenhower was open about the way he spoke. He didn't avoid speaking or try to cover up his difficulty. His non-fluent speech did not appear to distress him.

A noted psychologist, Joseph G. Sheehan, says that stuttering is like an iceberg. "The part above the surface, what people see and hear, is really the smaller part. By far the larger part is the part underneath—the shame, the fear, the guilt, all those other feelings that come to us when we try to speak a simple sentence and can't."

Stuttering was once considered by many to be a personality or emotional problem. It was thought to be a symptom of an underlying inner conflict, perhaps a sign that an individual had not successfully resolved some infantile need or desire.

Some psychologists today still believe that stuttering is a struggle between the need to go forward and the competing urge to hold back. You want to express yourself but are held back by fear. One thirteen-year-old stutterer says that talking for him is like Indian wrestling. He has to struggle constantly against his opponent (stuttering) so that it doesn't get the best of him.

Stuttering does seem to get worse under pressure and better when the pressure is removed. Most stutterers have hai dly any difficulty when they are relaxed. They do not usually stutter when they sing or talk to children or pets or to themselves out loud.

John Hammond, the blues singer, stutters when he speaks but not when he sings. "I first found I was free when I started to perform on stage," he told a reporter. "I was fifteen, I was in the school play, and I never stuttered." Both the movie star Marilyn Monroe and the television personality Garry Moore were stutterers before they became successful performers.

While some stutterers acquire neurotic behavior, stuttering is no longer generally thought to spring from deep-seated psychological problems. Therapists find that, as a group, stutterers are well adjusted. No important personality differences have been found between those who stutter and those who do not.

Stuttering is seen today mostly as a learned behavior that develops between the ages of two and five. This is the time when children are most actively acquiring speech and language. Experts who agree with this view say that all children stumble and hesitate during those years, perhaps because they are trying to adopt adult patterns of speech too quickly or because adults are pressuring them to speak fluently before they are ready or able.

Parents may create speech difficulties for a child by showing too much concern about normal hesitancies. A child who senses disapproval may try too hard to avoid repeating sounds or hesitating. This may make the child tense and anxious, even fearful. Constant corrections and interruptions may damage the child's fluency. A lack of interest or indifference to what the child is saying may have the same effect.

Heredity now appears to be another possible cause of stuttering. The disorder seems to run in families, like some other conditions that are passed on by the genes. About fifty percent of those who stutter have close relatives with a similar problem. If one identical twin stutters, there is a ninety percent chance that the other one does too. Still, it is not known how nor to what extent stuttering may be inherited. Much more research remains to be done.

Out of all the views on stuttering, the most recent is that stuttering is probably not caused by one but by several interacting factors. This view brings together the emotional problems that come from internal conflicts with possible physical factors, such as the body's timing of speech responses.

There may be a prolonged gap, for example, between what we say and what we hear ourselves say. This may show up in speech as stuttering. Embarrassment over the problem, perhaps combined with parental disapproval, may then make the condition worse.

Three complex sets of muscles are necessary for speech: the muscles used for breathing, those that control the larynx, and those that control the tongue, lips, and jaws. An imbalance in any of these muscles may trigger stuttering.

Until recently the outlook for those who stuttered was bleak. Only one-third of adult stutterers could improve significantly, a second third could improve somewhat, and

45

the rest could not improve at all. Now, pathologists are finding new ways to help stutterers. Whatever the cause, they say, most stutterers can overcome their problem by learning new ways of speaking.

OVERCOMING STUTTERING

There have been an amazing number of different treatments tried in the past to help people who stutter. Hundreds of stutterers had surgical operations to remove parts of their tongue. Large sums of money were spent on everything from mechanical devices that fit into the mouth to elaborate exercise regimens. Hypnosis was used, as well as individual and group therapy. Drugs, plus attempts to build up dominance on one side of the brain or the other, were also tried. None of these treatments was too successful.

Since people who stutter have difficulty controlling the muscles used for speech, many therapists are now focusing their attention on this aspect of the problem. They are training stutterers to unlearn certain physical responses to stressful situations. A variety of techniques are being used to help people develop new ways of breathing and controlling the larynx, tongue, lips, and jaws.

One method teaches stutterers to slow down their rate of speaking. Another teaches them to interrupt their speech when they feel trouble coming and to breathe deeply before starting to speak again. New York University's Martin F. Schwartz teaches individuals to sigh before speaking. The immediate cause of stuttering, he believes, is a locking of the vocal folds. The so-called airflow technique—taking a deep breath and letting air flow out during a conversation—helps a person who stutters to keep up the smooth flow of speech.

Some stutterers learn how to recognize and overcome a block when it is just beginning. The person is helped to realize that head jerks, grimaces, tongue clicks, postponement of feared words, and so on, do not help get the words out. In fact, they prevent the words from flowing. In some studies, speech training along with psychological counseling reduced stuttering in two-thirds of the cases after only a short period of treatment.

Most speech-language pathologists try to help patients change their basic attitudes and feelings about the way they speak. Stutterers who speak of their bodies as being in the hands of an enemy—"My lips refuse to open," or "My tongue gets in the way"—are helped to understand that they can do something about their condition.

One speech therapist gave this advice to a young man: "Those blocks may look and sound like monsters to you now, but you can turn them into straw men. Attack them. You must *refuse* to allow your words and fears to control you."

Stutterers who regard blocks with hostility and shame are often afraid to speak. This leads to still more stuttering. Most old therapies tried to eliminate the stuttering behavior. Most new therapies try to get rid of the fear. Stutterers are taught to bring their problem out into the open—talk more and avoid less.

Several novels contain stutterers as protagonists or heroes. Joseph Pillitteri's *Two Hours on Sunday* has as one of its principal characters a professional football coach who stutters; *The Revolution Script* by Brian Moore tells of a kidnapper-stutterer known as C.T. (Jacques Cosette-Trudel). One of the main characters of *Like Any Other Fugitive* by Joseph Hayes is a female stutterer. The Herman Wouk story, *The Winds of War,* describes what happened when the English author Somerset Maugham, who stuttered badly, met President Franklin Delano Roosevelt during World War II.

Several leading authorities on stuttering in recent years have themselves been stutterers. In fact, one estimate holds that more than fifty percent of those working in stuttering research have stuttering disorders. Although they vary in their views on the disorder, all the experts agree: Stutterers should admit to and confront their stuttering.

For years the distinguished professor of speech Charles Van Riper tried to keep from stuttering. His problem grew worse. He became fluent, he writes, only after he finally stopped trying to hide his problem.

How can you help a person who stutters? Here are some guides to follow:

• If someone is just beginning to stutter, ignore it.

• Don't call attention to the stutterer's problem. Overreaction can cause tension and lead to more stuttering.

• Be aware that professional help is available to overcome serious stuttering, but unless asked, do not suggest it directly to the person with a stutter.

• Don't tell the stutterer to relax or speak more slowly—don't make any such suggestions.

CHAPTER 7.

UNPLEASANT VOICES

POOR SPEAKING VOICES

Sally, aged twenty, always speaks in a soft, timid voice. It is sometimes hard to hear her and often difficult to understand what she is saying. Sally is always being asked to speak up, but as hard as she tries, there is almost never any real change in volume. Her doctor cannot find anything physically wrong with her.

For the last two years, sixteen-year-old Albert has been speaking in a high-pitched, falsetto voice that stays the same no matter what he is saying. Somewhat shy and overweight, Albert spends much more time at home than out with friends.

Eleven-year-old Barbara is the youngest in a family of seven children that all live together in a crowded apartment. Barbara often has to shout to be heard above the noise. Even when she is not at home, Barbara speaks with a rough, hoarse voice, as though she had a bad sore throat.

Sally, Albert, and Barbara all have voice disorders. Their voices are unintelligible or have an unpleasant effect on the listener.

About five percent of all school-aged children have voice disorders. But unlike articulation problems and stuttering, many voice disorders do not become evident until adolescence or adulthood.

Problems of loudness, or volume, make up one kind of voice disorder. The most frequent form of this disorder is speech that is too soft. In very severe cases, the person is not able to produce any sound at all, a condition called aphonia.

Some people have disorders related to pitch. They may speak in a pitch that is too high, that is too low, that never varies, or that varies inconsistently.

Other people have disorders of voice quality, or tone. They may speak in voices that are too strident (shrill) or raspy (harsh). Or, their voices may be breathy (weak and low-pitched), as if the person were suffering from asthma. A few sound hoarse (husky) and make you feel like clearing your own throat when you listen to them.

Occasionally you hear men and women with voices that are hypernasal (too resonant) or denasal (too little resonance). These people sound as though they have a head cold. Far too often, though, people with unpleasant voices have a combination of pitch, volume, and tonal problems.

Listen to the voices of your friends. See if you can recognize differences in volume. Do any of your friends' voices sound weak and nearly unintelligible? Do their voices rise and fall appropriately with what they are saying? Is the sound clear and pleasant?

Most adults and children need to pay more attention

to the sound of their voices. The human voice frequently needs training to serve as the wonderful tool of communication it is.

ABUSING OR
MISUSING THE VOICE

You will recall that when you speak, the sounds you make are produced by your vocal folds. The more air you force past the folds, the louder the sound; the less air, the softer the sound. Volume problems result when either too much or too little air is forced past the vocal folds.

People who always speak too loudly or too softly may have a hearing loss that prevents them from monitoring their own voices. Aphonia, the inability to produce sound, may result from an impaired larynx, caused by either organic damage or disease. Excessively soft speech, however, can also stem from psychological causes. The person may not want to be heard.

How high or how low your voice sounds depends on the length and tension of your vocal folds. When your larynx muscles shorten the folds, the pitch goes up; when the folds are lengthened, the pitch goes down. Pitch disorders usually result from too much or too little tension on the vocal folds. The cause may be a growth of some sort on the folds or the result of imitating poor speech models.

You have probably heard people, such as sidewalk hawkers, who have deliberately developed a grating, strident voice to attract attention. This kind of voice is usually caused by a strain in the larynx, which brings the vocal folds abnormally close together. People who are hostile and aggressive may develop strident voices as a result of tension. So do many teachers who strain to be heard above the noise in their classrooms.

Young adolescent boys sometimes develop rough or

raspy voices by trying to sound tough or very masculine. They may start by imitating a favorite movie star or some older boy. This lowering of the voice prematurely to sound older seldom causes permanent damage.

Almost everyone knows someone who speaks in a hoarse voice or in a voice that combines the qualities of breathiness and hoarseness. Hoarseness, while fairly common, is not terribly noticeable and is often the result of overuse or abuse of the voice, which causes the vocal folds to become thick and swollen. Occasionally it is a sign of growths on the larynx.

Dysphonia refers to any disturbance in voice production. One of the most extreme voice problems is a condition known as spastic dysphonia. In spastic dysphonia, a tightness of the vocal folds and often of the whole vocal system interferes with speech. A person with spastic dysphonia can speak at times, but the voice sounds harsh and strained. Sometimes the problem is related to an organic disorder, such as paralysis, that affects the larynx. More often it comes from serious emotional difficulties.

Have you ever heard someone use a high-pitched, nasal voice to make fun of another person's speech? The sound is made by creating more than normal resonance in the nose. Some people always speak this way. It is called hypernasality. This disorder may be due to air passing through an abnormal opening between the throat and the nasal cavity. Sometimes air leaks through a space in the palate, the bone and tissue structure that separates the top of the mouth from the nose. Hypernasality is often found in people who are born with cleft lip and palate. It is also found in people who are low in vitality or who are in the habit of using a whining voice to get sympathy from others.

When you have a head cold, your voice almost always sounds different than usual. This "cold-in-the-head" quality, also called denasality or hyponasality, is the opposite of hypernasality. It results when the sound waves carried by the air do not pass through the nose at all, and there is little or no nasal resonance. Clamp your fingers over your nostrils and say, "Spring has come." Do you hear how dull and congested your voice sounds? The words sound more like "Sprig has cub." That is because the /g/ and /b/ sounds are substituted for the nasal sounds /ng/ and /m/. The usual causes are obstructions due to enlarged adenoids, nasal congestion, an infection, or growths.

As you can see, voice disorders have many causes. In most people, however, unpleasant or unintelligible speech is the result of some abuse or misuse of the body's speech mechanism. Disorders of volume, pitch, and tone can almost always be overcome with the help of a speech specialist.

TREATING VOICE DISORDERS

Almost all of us are capable of developing more pleasant voices than the ones we have. Although it is not easy, it is never too late to modify the sound of your voice.

Tape recorders are a good way to help you improve the way you sound. Record and then listen carefully to some samples of your speech. How do you think you sound?

If you want to improve your voice, make daily recordings. Experiment with varying pitch, volume, and tone until you achieve a more pleasant sound. Then practice whenever you can. Every time you sit down at the dinner table, for example, concentrate on your voice. Eventually, you will find yourself using your "new" voice in all situations.

Most therapists follow the same three basic steps

in teaching voice improvement. The first step involves discovering the cause or abuse that led to the problem. The second step is to eliminate the cause and minimize the abuse. And lastly, the therapist helps the person to find his or her best voice.

Sarah, a twenty-one-year-old college student, spoke in a throaty voice that sounded very affected and snobbish. Before treatment began, the therapist tried to learn as much as he could about her speech history. When did she begin to speak this way? Was the disorder the result of an accident or illness? Were there any serious psychological problems? Did the problem develop through imitation of others?

The exam did not turn up either a physical or a psychological problem. Therefore, instead of referring Sarah to a physician or psychologist, the therapist listened very carefully, sometimes with special instruments, to the volume, pitch, and resonance of Sarah's speaking voice. He judged her potential for voice improvement, then discussed his goals with her and planned a course of treatment.

In Sarah's case, the goal was to modify her usual way of speaking. She was taught special exercises for her larynx and given breathing-improvement exercises, ear training, and vocal training.

Voice disorders like Sarah's may be caused by insufficient breath supply or by irregular breath flow. Sarah was therefore taught to become aware of her breathing patterns and also shown how to control her breath stream. In addition, the therapist helped her to find her best pitch level and to hear the faults in her own speech. Once Sarah focused on her voice problems, she started improving.

Sarah acquired a new speaking voice and was helped to use it in day-to-day speech. She hopes now that she will do better in college and be successful in the law career she intends to pursue.

Some disorders, of course, are so serious that they require surgery or medication before voice therapy can begin. Often the surgical removal of tumors or other growths will improve the ability of the vocal folds to vibrate. Certain drugs may help the voice by reducing swelling in the folds.

About ten thousand Americans each year undergo operations for larynx cancer, a cancer frequently associated with smoking. In one procedure, the surgeon removes the larynx, then connects the trachea to a hole cut in the patient's neck for breathing.

To talk again, the person may be taught esophageal speech. The therapist shows the patient how to form words while swallowing air and expelling it. This produces a low-pitched, eerie sort of voice that only half of the patients are able to master.

Another approach uses an artificial larynx, also called an electrolarynx. A vibrating diaphragm as the basic sound source is held just under the chin. Then, by manipulating tongue, lips, and jaws, the user is able to make the sounds of speech. In another type of device, air from the trachea is directed through tubing and past a vibrating reed to produce the basic sounds, which the person then forms into speech.

People who have lost their natural voices because of surgery or some other cause often join the International Association of Laryngectomees (IAL) or a local branch of the Lost Chords or New Voice clubs, to meet others with the same problem and receive the latest information.

Damage to the brain or spinal cord, due to cerebral palsy, stroke, or some other illness, can make both walking *and* talking impossible for some patients. A new invention called the "talking wheelchair," which is part wheelchair and part computer, is letting many of these patients speak for the first time. It works this way: On the lap tray of the wheelchair is a board with squares. Each square is marked with a letter, word, or complete sentence. The user moves a pointer to a square, and the computer that is built into the board produces the sound of the letter, word, or sentence on that square. This so-called synthesized speech, made possible by computers, offers many exciting possibilities for people with severe speech disorders.

To review, here are some signs of a vocal disorder:
- A person has continuous or recurring hoarseness.
- A person's voice is too low or too high for his or her sex.
- A person tries to sound like some actress, actor, or other model, rather than speak in a normal voice.
- A person is often criticized for speaking too softly or too loudly.
- A person has had several temporary losses of voice.

CHAPTER 8.

LANGUAGE DIFFICULTIES

LANGUAGE-LEARNING PROBLEMS

Kim seemed to develop normally for the first two years of her life. Then, sometime after her second birthday, problems began to appear. Although healthy in all other respects, Kim barely spoke. She was unable to ask for anything; she could not remember the names of members of her family. Neither did she seem to understand what others said to her. She became irritable, demanding, and restless.

Although her parents were concerned, they did not seek help. They believed that Kim would outgrow these difficulties.

When she was five-and-a-half years old, Kim entered kindergarten. Her teacher soon recognized the symptoms. Kim was suffering from a language disorder. This is a general term used to describe any problem in which there is difficulty expressing or understanding language. Kim was given special help to overcome her academic and behavior problems. She also began to receive speech therapy.

Now, at age ten, Kim is beginning to speak. She still has many difficulties with articulation and with putting words together into sentences. She understands only the simplest speech of others. Her problems continue in the area of social adjustment. Although Kim will probably never speak normally, she will be able to communicate with short sentences and a limited vocabulary.

People with language disorders fall into three groups: those who fail to acquire any language, those who are delayed in acquiring language, and those who lose language due to brain injury, accident, or disease. Language-learning problems vary widely. They include an inability to store or recall sound patterns or meanings and difficulty in putting ideas into words. Estimates of how many people suffer from these problems vary greatly too. The U.S. Department of Education puts the figure of children with language disorders at 8.7 million.

Four-year-old Johnny didn't speak any better than a two-year-old. Whenever he tried to say something, he would become frustrated. His parents could not understand the sounds he made. Children in the neighborhood didn't want to play with him because he could not communicate with them.

Johnny was becoming very difficult to live with. He insisted on constant attention and was overactive and very hard to discipline. His mother thought that his problem was psychological, that he was jealous of the attention his baby sister was getting.

She was wrong. An examination by a speech-language pathologist showed that Johnny's hearing was normal, but that he confused the sounds of speech.

Johnny could not tell /b/ from /d/. *Bad* and *dad* sounded the same to him. This confusion with sounds led to his poor articulation. He reversed syllables and omitted or substituted some consonants. When he said, "Bah too ma tuh bah goo," he meant, "Daddy took me to buy gum."

The examiner also found that Johnny had a poor memory for sounds. He could not remember the names of objects or recall words that he had learned. When given two digits—"two, three," for example—Johnny could say them back. But when it came to recalling three digits—"two, three, one"—Johnny said "two, three," and after a very long pause, "two?" He seemed disobedient, but in fact he simply could not remember directions long enough to follow them through.

Johnny's problem with language is called a learning disability. Doctors say that he has an immature nervous system, or that he suffers from minimal brain dysfunction. His problems stem from some disorder in the pathways that carry messages from his sense organs to his brain. The messages he gets become jumbled and confused. That is why he can't make sense of what his ears hear, even though his hearing is fine.

Some children are born with autism, an inability to relate to people and social situations in a normal way. From the very start, the child does not respond to its mother and seems to be out of touch with the world. The baby may cry all the time or be unusually quiet. From age one on, autistic children spend much of their time rocking back and forth, flapping their hands, or simply staring. They often find it hard to understand speech and may not speak at all. Others imitate what they hear without seeming to understand what they are saying.

Among children who are sometimes diagnosed as

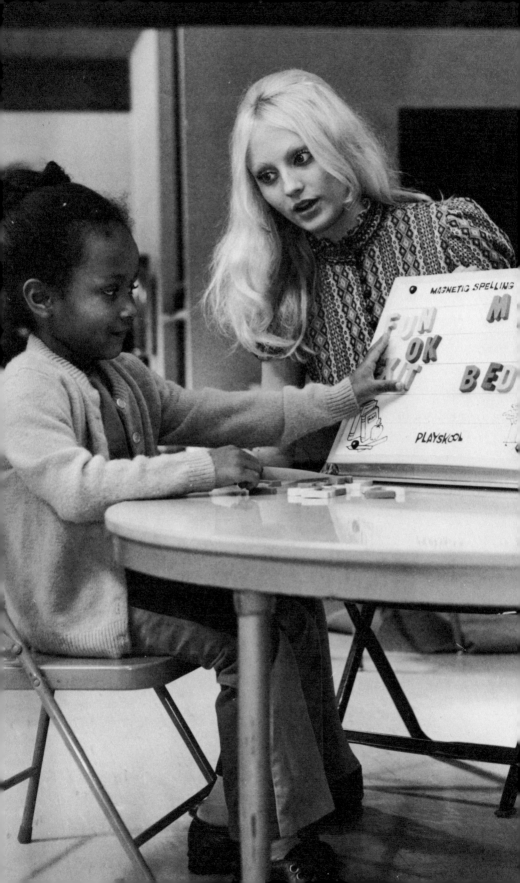

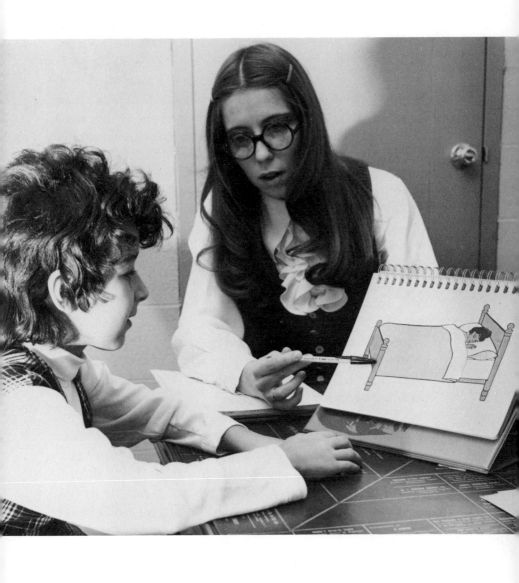

*Since there is such a wide range of
language-learning problems, a variety of
treatment strategies is used.*

autistic are those who instead have childhood aphasia, also called congenital aphasia. In childhood aphasia there is a failure to acquire language. Aphasic children have a normal year or two of life but are slow to acquire speech or language. Most do not even begin to talk until around age three or four. Childhood aphasia is usually defined as the failure of otherwise normal children to develop, or to develop by normal means, speech and language. Aphasic children may eventually be able to speak in sentences, but in general they remain better able to understand language than to produce it.

Aphasia in adults is different from childhood aphasia. Adult aphasia is the loss of language and may result from a stroke, a blockage of blood in an artery of the brain. It can also be caused by a brain injury, such as from a gunshot wound or severe blow to the head, or a brain tumor. People who develop aphasia are struck by an inability to use words properly or appropriately. They may have trouble in both expressing and understanding speech.

The children with language-learning problems in the examples we have considered have normal or above-normal intelligence. But something happened to them before, during, or after birth to cause their problems. Birth injury, exposure of the pregnant mother to viral disease or drugs, severe head injuries—all can lead to language difficulties in children. But everyone agrees that, whatever the cause, the end result is some interference in the functioning of the brain and nervous system.

Impaired development in language often accompanies mental retardation. Children with limited intellectual ability are likely to have some degree of difficulty in understanding speech and in speaking. The extent of these problems usually depends on the severity of the retardation. Profoundly retarded children usually have little or no ability to use language. Less severely retarded people may be just below average in their language skills.

Of course, hearing loss in children results in multiple problems in the area of speech and language development. (See Chapter 7.) Difficulty in hearing the speech of others and the sound of one's own voice almost always leads to problems in mastering language.

DIAGNOSTIC TEACHING

Seldom is the exact cause of a language-learning problem known. Yet most of these disorders can be helped. Many parents, when they realize that their child is not talking or is talking at a level below others of the same age, take the youngster to a speech-language expert.

The therapist usually interviews the parents and the child and then uses various language tests to diagnose the disorder. The purpose is not to put a label on the child but to decide on the approach that will work best. When necessary, the therapist turns to another specialist—an audiologist, a pediatrician, a neurologist, a psychologist, or a psychiatrist—before reaching a conclusion.

Based on the diagnosis, the therapist chooses a set of strategies. The idea is to build on the person's particular strengths and eliminate the areas of weakness. Each person's problems are different. Therefore, each approach has to be individual. The strategy that is used depends on where the difficulty lies and which approach will work best. This method of combining diagnosis with therapy is called diagnostic teaching.

Recently a therapist had her first meeting with Sally, a thin, frightened-looking child who did not speak at all. The speech teacher talked as little as possible. She tried to get down to Sally's own level of communication and establish a relationship that would make the girl want to

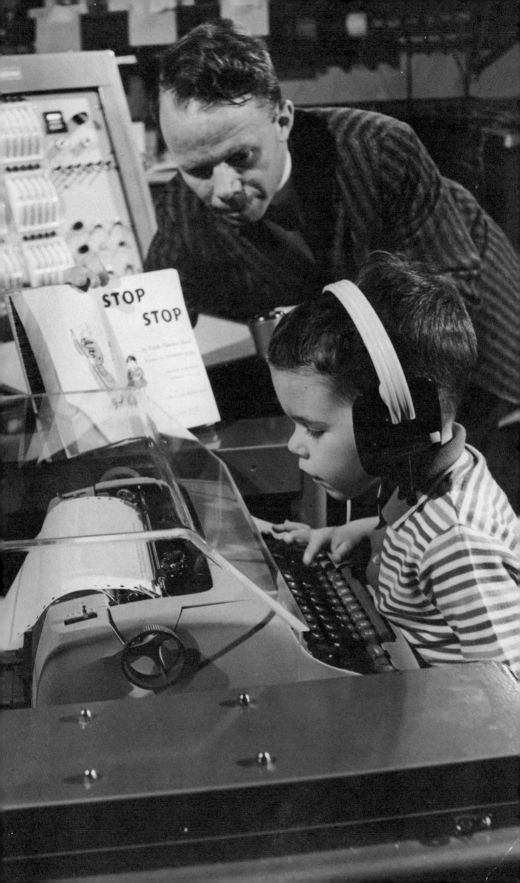

talk. The therapist also performed a number of repetitive actions. She banged on a drum, clapped her hands, and bounced up and down. She encouraged Sally to imitate her.

Once Sally was used to the play activity, the therapist introduced talk into the sessions. She hoped that Sally would imitate her speech and language as she had imitated her gestures. First the therapist made noises, then she said single words, then short phrases, and finally sentences. Sally was helped to follow the speech patterns. The therapist's speech became the model for Sally to express her own thoughts and to discover that talking is useful.

Many therapists use operant conditioning to achieve language mastery. This method is one of many possible strategies. The basic idea is to build toward a goal by moving through a series of small, controlled steps. The child receives positive reinforcement at each step along the way. The reinforcement for performing the desired behavior might be a hug, a smile, a small reward, or credit toward a prize.

Let's say that the therapist's goal with a nonverbal child like Sally is to get her to make sounds. Each time the child does make a sound, for example says ''boo,''

"Talking typewriters," such as this one developed by Westinghouse Research Laboratories, provide individual attention plus reinforcement every step of the way. Here, as the child types out a word, the machine says it aloud with the correct pronunciation and then spells it.

the therapist repeats the sound and smiles at the child. To help the child remember the sound, the teacher says a word such as "boot," which uses that sound. She then helps the child to learn the word by showing her a picture of a boot or placing a boot in her hands.

When the child seems ready, the teacher may try to get him or her to form short phrases. She'll say, "Want boot" while taking the boot away from the child. The child gets the boot back when he or she tries to say the phrase. Eventually the child's vocabulary starts to grow. He or she forms new words and phrases.

From the start, the parents are taught how to stimulate the child to talk at home. The therapist tries to relieve the parents' fears and worries. As the adults become more positive in their attitudes, they create better conditions at home for the child to acquire language.

It may take months or years, but gradually Sally will talk more often. She will come to rely less on gestures for communication and more on words. More important, Sally will begin to feel less frustrated and thus less tense and unhappy.

Children with poor speech and language due to faulty models at home or a deprived environment, and those with learning disabilities, usually make the best progress under treatment. Aphasic children, autistic children, and children who are mentally retarded generally make slower progress and usually need treatment for a longer period of time. The most severe cases may never develop satisfactory speech or language.

Diagnosis and therapy are very important for all who have language disorders. Ignoring such difficulties can only create additional problems for the individual. What language-disordered people need most are lots of stimulating activities and encouragement to improve their communication skills.

To review, here are some signs of language disorders:

- A person speaks less and has a much smaller vocabulary than others of the same age.
- A person cannot say what he or she needs or wants as well as most others of the same age.
- A person cannot express his or her ideas.
- A person cannot understand or respond appropriately to what is being said.
- A person does not use language to learn and to ask about things he or she does not understand.

CHAPTER 9.

MULTIPLE DIFFICULTIES

HEARING LOSS

No matter how intelligent you are or how eager you are to learn, if you cannot hear you will have trouble talking. When you cannot hear what is said to you, you cannot learn what sounds mean or how to imitate the sounds that others make.

Different kinds of damage to the ear cause different hearing problems. The most common kind of hearing impairment is conductive loss. This hearing loss results from damage to the outer or middle ear. Such damage, either present at birth or caused by accident or disease, interferes with the passage of sounds and vibrations to the inner ear.

Soon after she was born, Debbie showed signs of conductive hearing loss. Her parents noticed that she was not startled by sudden or loud noises. She did not turn her head at the sound of a familiar voice. She did not imitate the sounds her parents made. Although Debbie did babble for a short while, the babbling stopped at about seven months.

By one year, Debbie still did not respond to being called or to household sounds. At two, she spoke only a few words. By the time she was three, she could put some words together but her articulation was very poor.

Physical exams and audiometric tests showed that Debbie had been born with very narrow auditory canals in her outer ears. Almost no sound was able to get through to her inner ears. She could hear sounds only if they were very loud and had been produced 3 feet (.9 m) or less from her.

In conductive loss, individuals hear sounds as muffled and soft. Only if the sounds are very loud can the person with conductive loss hear them clearly.

Among all the children in the United States, about one million have significant hearing handicaps. About eighty percent have conductive loss like Debbie's. This kind of loss can be helped most.

Debbie was helped to hear better by being fit with a hearing aid. The device amplifies sounds and directs them through the bones of the head to the inner ear. Once the sounds are made louder, the person can hear quite well. Debbie will probably always substitute or omit some sounds when speaking, though. Her voice will tend to be nasal, high-pitched, and monotonous. But she will be able to speak and communicate with others.

Sometimes infections from sore throats spread into the middle ear and block off the chamber so that air cannot get in. Too much air pressure on the other side of the eardrum can cause the membrane to rupture and be permanently damaged.

Doctors therefore prescribe antibiotics to treat infections in the early stages. By treating an illness before it becomes serious, it is frequently possible to prevent this kind of hearing loss.

A far less common but much more serious type of hearing impairment is sensori-neural loss. A few years ago, a team of physicians and speech-language pathologists examined a child named Bobby. His teachers and parents considered Bobby emotionally disturbed. The experts, though, found that he had a sensori-neural hearing loss.

For Bobby, the damage was not in his outer or middle ear. It was in his inner ear, where sound frequencies stimulate the nerve cells in the cochlea. Damage to these cells, or to the pathways that lead to the brain, cause difficulty in hearing certain sounds.

Like others with this kind of loss, Bobby could hear some sounds very well but others not at all. Because he heard incompletely, he could not understand what he heard. This is what made his behavior so puzzling to the adults around him.

Bobby heard the high-pitched sounds but missed the low-pitched ones. Others with this kind of loss may hear the low sounds but not the high ones. And for some, where there is extensive damage to the cochlea, all sounds are blocked out.

Many times the damage that results in sensori-neural loss occurs before the child is born. The inner ear and its nerve pathways do not develop properly. Or,

Sign language is learned by many hearing-impaired people, though a large number also use speech to communicate.

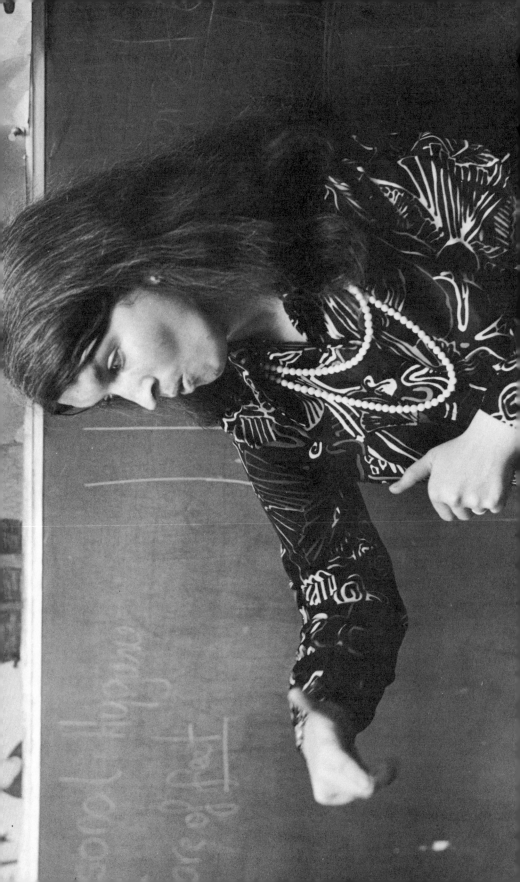

the mother contracts German measles, flu, or mumps during pregnancy, which may cause nerve damage in the newborn. Serious diseases during childhood, such as scarlet fever or meningitis, can also cause nerve damage.

Once a nerve cell is damaged, its function cannot be restored. Hearing aids may help in cases of mild or moderate sensori-neural loss by amplifying sounds. But training in lip-reading, and in sign language as well, is almost always needed to help the child develop an ability to communicate. With the right kind of help, most acquire enough speech and language to be able to attend a regular school.

CEREBRAL PALSY

Billy has cerebral palsy. He is now eighteen years old and a sophomore in high school. Although Billy can function as well as his friends in some areas, his speech is quite hard to understand.

Billy's problem stems from his inability to move or control his lips, jaws, and tongue. He will always slur his words and have poor articulation, but speech therapy is making his speech more fluent, stronger, and more understandable.

Cerebral palsy is a general term for a group of conditions that result from damage to the brain, especially those areas of the brain that control the body's muscles. Since the brain directs the movements that make speech possible, any problem associated with it will make talking very difficult.

Cerebral palsy usually results from an injury to the brain or spinal cord before, during, or after birth. The injury may be great or slight. The condition does not usually worsen, nor does it go away in time. About seventy percent of those with cerebral palsy have articulation problems, often accompanied by fluency, voice, and language difficulties as well. Hearing loss, usually in the high-frequency range, occurs in about twenty percent of all cases.

In the spastic form of cerebral palsy, the muscles overcontract; they pull too suddenly and too hard. This makes the smooth or gradual muscle movements needed for speech very difficult. Speech sounds explode out or come out sounding blurred. Lack of muscular control also means that lip and tongue movements are hard to make. If, for example, the tongue cannot touch the upper gum ridge, it is almost impossible to produce the /t/, /d/, and /n/ sounds.

Involuntary contractions of the muscles in people with cerebral palsy cause twitching or uncontrolled shaking and can affect any part of the body. When this kind of cerebral palsy, called athetoid, affects the face, it greatly impairs speech. Breathing problems often make words sound no louder than a whisper. The voice shakes and is of poor quality, with uneven pitch.

The lack of muscle control caused by cerebral palsy delays the development of speech. The lack of mobility and slowness in developing skills may result in babying by parents and limited life experiences. Because people with cerebral palsy often spend much of their time alone, they sometimes need extra help in learning to communicate with others. The difficulties in speaking clearly and learning skills can lead to tension and further aggravate the problems the person with cerebral palsy has to face.

Those most severely afflicted with cerebral palsy may be completely unable to speak. They can learn to communicate, though, by using so-called conversation boards. These boards are similar to the boards used in the talking wheelchairs. They have pictures of common objects in each square. The person points to the objects or words to make himself or herself understood. Others talk back in the same way. This kind of communication, in an atmosphere of love and caring, helps overcome even the most difficult of problems.

CLEFT PALATE AND LIP

Mike, now ten, was born with a cleft palate and lip, an opening in the roof of his mouth that extended forward, leaving a space in his upper lip as well. At ages two and four, Mike had operations to close the openings in his palate and lip. After the surgery, Mike worked with a speech-language pathologist. His parents helped him to do certain training exercises at home. By the time he entered school, Mike's speech difficulties and the cleft itself were hardly noticeable.

Slightly more than one out of every thousand infants born in the United States have a cleft of some sort. A cleft lip is a lip that is separated into two or three parts. Usually the cleft is through the skin, muscle, and inner membrane of the upper lip. Occasionally it may instead involve the lower part of the lip, or go all the way up to the nostril. A cleft palate may affect only the soft palate or both the soft and hard palates.

A cleft lip is usually the result of some deviation in the development of the face during the second month of prenatal growth. A cleft palate may be caused by some interference with the formation of the palate, usually during the third month of prenatal development.

Some doctors suspect that radiation, drugs, or certain chemicals may cause the condition. Others think it may be due to a failure of the tongue to drop out of the way in time for the space to close, or that some defect in the chromosomes may be responsible.

Cleft lip occurs about twice as often among males as females; cleft palate is just the opposite. There are some families in which children with clefts are born in every

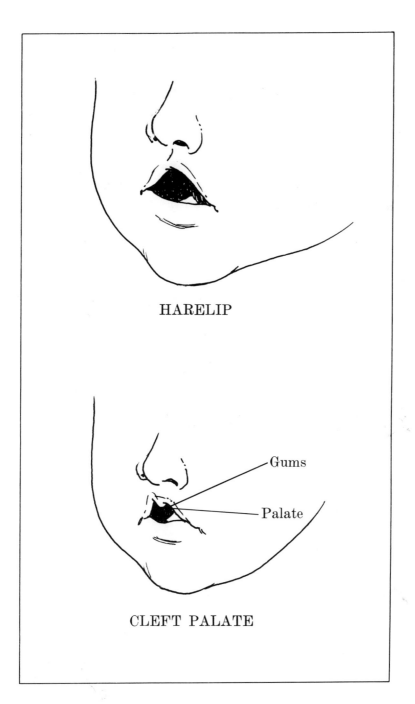

HARELIP

Gums

Palate

CLEFT PALATE

generation. But in most cases, there is no history of clefts in the family.

Because of his cleft lip and palate, Mike had the most trouble producing the consonant sounds /p/, /t/, /s/, and /sh/. When speech treatment began, Mike could not make his tongue move more than a fraction of an inch in any direction.

Also, as in others with cleft palates, the soft palate and the throat did not work together as they do in normal speech. They did not close off the passage between the mouth and the nose during the production of most sounds. Air passed through the cleft into the nose. This produced unwanted resonance, making the voice hypernasal.

The first thing that Mike's speech teacher taught him was how to control his breathing and develop enough air pressure for speaking. He had to learn which sounds required him to send air through his nose and which did not.

Mike's training started with words that included the consonant sounds he could make. This led to instruction on new sounds that were more difficult for him to produce. It took several years of help, but Mike eventually learned to speak quite clearly.

There is no single treatment for children who have clefts. Clefts of the palate often require surgery, the use of a molded plastic appliance to cover the opening between the nose and throat, or both. Quite often, there is a need for speech therapy as well.

Like most speech-disordered individuals, the vast majority of people with clefts can achieve normal or near-normal speech and language. Early diagnosis, careful training, and loving concern from family members, teachers, and friends are the ingredients for success.

GLOSSARY

Aphasia—Loss of language function due to brain damage.

Aphonia—Loss of voice due to functional or organic difficulty.

Articulation—Adjustments and movements of speech organs to produce all the sounds of speech.

Articulators—Structures involved in the production of the sounds of speech.

Athetoid—A form of cerebral palsy characterized by marked tremors or uncontrolled shaking.

Audiologist—A specialist trained to evaluate and help people with hearing problems.

Audiometer—A machine for gauging the ability of an individual to hear.

Autism—A disorder characterized by language difficulties and almost complete withdrawal.

Babbling—A stage in vocal development involving non-meaningful combinations of sounds.

Block—A sudden difficulty in speaking experienced by a person trying to talk.

Cerebral Palsy—A general term for a group of disorders that affects the body's muscle control.

Cleft Lip—A congenital separation of the upper lip into two or three parts.

Cleft Palate—A congenital defect in which there is an opening in the roof of the mouth.

Communication—Transfer of information between individuals by any means.

Conductive Hearing Loss—The most common kind of hearing loss; caused by damage to the outer or middle ear.

Congenital—Existing at or dating from birth.

Cooing—A stage in vocal development involving pleasure sounds.

Delayed Language—Slowness in the development of language skills needed to express and understand thoughts and ideas.

Denasality—Too little resonance in the nose, causing in the voice a stuffy, "cold-in-the-head" quality.

Diagnostic Teaching—Remedial work, carried on individually or in small groups, that is based on evaluation and information gathered from professional sources.

Dysphonia—Any disturbance of voice production.

Eardrum—See *Tympanic Membrane*.

Esophageal Speech—A way of speaking for people who have lost the use of their larynx.

Fluency—The ability to speak without frequent interruptions or hesitations; smooth, flowing speech.

Functional Disorder—A disorder without a known physical cause.

Hearing—The sense that receives sound.

Hearing Aid—A device that is worn to amplify sound in order to improve hearing.

Hypernasality—Too much resonance in the nose, giving the voice a nasal quality.

Jargon—A type of vocal play in babies in which utterances consist of meaningless sounds.

Lallation—A stage in language development in which the baby repeats syllables.

Language—The ability to use speech sounds to express one's thoughts and emotions.

Laryngitis—An inflammation of the tissues of the larynx that causes hoarseness at first, then temporary loss of the voice if the condition persists.

Larynx—The "voice box"; contains the vocal folds whose vibrations produce sound.

Learning Disabilities—Difficulties in receiving information from the messages that are taken in through the senses.

Lisping—Defective articulation of certain sounds by substitution of other sounds.

Loudness—Perception of sound according to the intensity or energy of that sound.

Operant Conditioning—A system of rewards given for making the correct response. For example, a child makes a sound correctly and is given a candy.

Organic Disorder—A disorder caused by a physical or structural impairment.

Palate—Hard or soft palate; the roof of the mouth separating the mouth from the nasal cavity. Made of bone and tissue.

Pharynx—The passageway above the larynx that leads to the mouth and the nose.

Pitch—A property of sound—its highness or lowness—

determined by the frequency of the sound waves.

Psychologist—A person trained to treat behavioral or emotional problems.

Resonators—Structures in the vocal tract that amplify the vocal sound coming from the larynx.

Sensori-Neural Hearing Loss—Damage in the inner ear or in the pathways to the brain.

Spastic—The form of cerebral palsy in which the muscles overcontract.

Speech—The ability to produce sounds.

Speech-Language Pathologist—A specialist engaged in the study of speech and language disorders.

Stroke—A blockage or hemorrhage in an artery of the brain that may affect the ability to communicate with language.

Stuttering—An interruption in the flow or rhythm of speech.

Synthesized Speech—Speech that is electronically produced by a computer.

Tympanic Membrane—The tissue that separates the middle and outer ear. Also called the eardrum.

Vocal Folds—Also called vocal cords; two small bands of tissue that vibrate and, when stimulated by the passage of air, produce sound.

Voice Box—See *Larynx*.

Volume—Degree of loudness or softness of a sound.

SPEECH ORGANIZATIONS

If you wish further information on speech
or speech disorders, you may write:

*The National Association for
Hearing and Speech Action*
6110 Executive Blvd., Suite 1000
Rockville, Maryland 20852

American Speech-Language-Hearing Association
10801 Rockville Pike, Rockville, Maryland 20852

*The Alexander Graham Bell Association
for the Deaf, Inc.*
3417 Volta Place, N.W., Washington, D.C. 20007

*National Institute of Neurological and
Communicative Disorders and Stroke*
National Institutes of Health
9000 Rockville Pike, Rockville, Maryland 20852

BIBLIOGRAPHY

Karlin, Isaac W. *Development and Disorders of Speech in Childhood*. Springfield, Ill.: Charles C. Thomas Publishers, 1977.

Molloy, Julia S. *Teaching the Retarded Child to Talk: A Guide for Parents and Teachers*. New York: John Day Company, 1961.

Travis, Lee Edward. *Handbook of Speech Pathology and Audiology*. Englewood, Cliffs, N.J.: Prentice-Hall, 1971.

Van Riper, Charles. *Speech Correction: Principles and Methods*. 5th edition. Englewood Cliffs, N.J.: Prentice-Hall, 1972.

SUGGESTED READING

Browning, Elizabeth. *I Can't See What You Are Saying.* New York: Coward, McCann & Geoghegan, 1973. (The story of Freddy Browning, a partially deaf and almost totally aphasic child, and his parents' difficulties in finding proper care and treatment for his disabilities.)

Cameron, Constance Carpenter. *A Different Drum.* Englewood Cliffs, New Jersey: Prentice-Hall, Inc., 1973. (Describes a mother's efforts to meet the needs of her aphasic son.)

Charlip, Remy, and Mary Beth. *Handtalk: An ABC of Finger Spelling and Sign Language.* New York: Parents Magazine Press, 1974. (Teaches the reader how to communicate through sign language and finger spelling.)

Greenfield, Josh. *A Child Called Noah.* New York: Holt, Rinehart, and Winston, 1972. (A diary written by the father of an autistic child.)

Kastein, Shulamith, and Trace, Barbara. *The Birth of Language: The Case History of a Non-Verbal Child.* Springfield, Illinois: Charles C. Thomas Publishers, 1970. (A mother and a speech therapist tell of their work with Joan, a child who had speech and language impairments.)

Lash, Joseph P. *Helen and Teacher.* New York: Delacorte/Seymour Lawrence, 1980. (A modern version of the Helen Keller story.)

Levine, Edna S. *Lisa and Her Soundless World.* New York: Human Sciences Press, 1974. (The story of Lisa shows what it is like to be hearing-impaired. Explains treatment techniques, lip reading, and finger spelling.)

Moore, Brian. *The Revolution Script.* New York: Holt, Rinehart, and Winston, 1971. (Tells of a kidnapper-stutterer known as C.T.)

Pillitteri, Joseph. *Two Hours on Sunday.* New York: Dial Press, 1971. (One of the principal characters in this novel is a professional football coach who stutters.)

INDEX

Airflow technique, 46
Amplifying equipment, 14
Antibiotics, 69–70
Anvil, 16
Apes, and speech, 2–5
Aphasia, 62, 77
Aphonia, 50, 51, 77
Articulation, 77; disorders of, 8–9, 30, 32–34
Articulators, 14, 77
Athetoid, 73, 77
Audiologist, 34, 77
Audiometer, 34, 35, 77
Auditory nerve, 16
Autism, 59, 62, 77

Babbling, 22, 24–25, 78
Bigart, Homer, 42
Block, 47, 78
Brain, and sound, 16, 18; and speech, 4
Brain dysfunction, 59
Breathing, 54

Cerebral palsy, 34, 72–74, 78; spastic form of, 73
Chest, 14
Cleft lip, 52, 74–76, 78
Cleft palate, 52, 74–76, 78
Cochlea, 16, 70
Communication, 2, 4, 6, 19, 78

Conductive hearing loss, 68, 78
Congenital, 78
Conversation boards, 73–74
Cooing, 23–25, 78
Crying, 22, 23–24

Delayed language, 18, 78
Denasality, 53, 78
Diagnostic teaching, 63, 65–66, 78
Dysphonia, 52, 78

Eardrum, 16, 78
Electrolarynx, 55
Errors of omission, 32
Esophageal speech, 55, 77

First words, 26–27
Fluency, 78
Functional speech disorder, 33, 78

Gestures, 25–26

Hammer, 16
Hammond, John, 44
Hearing, 14, 16–17, 79
Hearing aids, 69, 72, 79
Hearing centers, 16
Hoarseness, 52
Hypernasality, 52, 79

Inner ear, 16, 70; fluid in, 16

International Association of Laryngectomees (IAL), 55

Jargon, 27, 79
Jaws, 14

Lallation, 24–25, 79
Language, 6, 10, 79; development, 20; difficulties, 57–67; disorders, 9, 18, 57–58, 67; learning problems, 57–63
Larynx, 13–14, 79; cancer of, 55; laryngitis, 79
Learning disability, 59, 79
Lips, 14
Lisp, 32, 79
Lost Chords club, 55
Loudness, 9, 50, 79. *See also* Volume

Memory center, 18
Mental retardation, 62–63
Middle ear, 16
Mouth, 14
Multiple difficulties, 68–76

Nerve pathways, 18
New Voice club, 55
Nose, 14

Operant conditioning, 39, 79
Organic speech disorder, 33, 79
Oval window, 16

Palate, 52, 79
Pharynx, 14, 79
Pitch, 79–80; problems, 50–51
Prehistoric civilizations, and speech, 1–2
Psychologist, 36, 44, 63, 80

Religion, and communication, 2
Repeating words, 22
Resonators, 14, 80

Schwartz, Martin F., 46
Sensori-neural hearing loss, 70, 72, 80
Sensory-motor approach to speech therapy, 39
Shuhan, Joseph G., 43
Sinuses, 14
Soft palate, 14
Sound, as electrical code, 16; interpretation of, 16, 18–20; production, 13–14; and words, 22–29
Spastic, 80
Spastic dysphonia, 52
Speech, 10, 13–15, 80; blocks, 47; disturbances, 20; errors, 30–40; faulty learning, 34, 36; origins of, 1–6; rhythm, 78; sound distortions, 32–33; therapy, 36, 39–40
Speech and language disorders, 7–9, 11–13, 20–21

Speech-language pathologists, 20, 33, 80
Stirrup, 16
Stroke, 55, 62, 80
Stutterers, 9; as protagonists in novels, 47–48
Stuttering, 41–48, 80
Substitution mistake, 32
Synthesized speech, 56, 80

Talking, learning how, 22
Talking typewriters, 2, 64
Talking wheelchair, 55–56, 73
Tape recorders, 31, 53
Templin-Darley Articulation Tests, 34
Throat, 14
Tone, 50
Tongue, 14
Tympanic membrane, 80. *See also* Eardrum

Van Riper, Charles, 48
Vibrating diaphragm, 55
Vibrations, 14, 16
Vocal chords, 13–14. *See also* Vocal folds
Vocal folds, 51
Voice, abuse of, 51; disorders, 9, 49–56
Voice box, 13, 80. *See also* **Larynx**
Volume, 50, 80

Windpipe, 13
Words into sentences, 27–29

ABOUT
THE AUTHOR

Gilda Berger, a one-time teacher in the area of special education, has previously authored books for Franklin Watts on the subjects of learning disabilities, physical disabilities, and the gifted and talented. She is currently at work on a book about mental illness.

Gilda is married to author Melvin Berger. They have two daughters and live in Great Neck, Long Island (N.Y.).